Eye and eyelash diseases and disorders

Chrysalis House Publishing

Eye and eyelash diseases and disorders
Copyright © 2014 by Chrysalis House Publishing

Chrysalis House Publishing
Louise Prunty
Lower Ground
7 Newton Place
Glasgow
G3 7PR
United Kingdom

publishinguk@me.com
www.chrysalishousepublishing.com

Contents

Foreword

The human eye is arguably our most important sensory organ, its complexity fitting of the function it performs. Many texts exist focusing on individual components of the eye and of course many professional bodies, such as optometrists and ophthalmologists are responsible for looking after our sight. It is easy to get lost in the mass of information relating to the eye and its important surrounding structures.

What is needed is a concise summary of the relevant points, in addition what and where things can go wrong. In my opinion a solid knowledge base on which to build is key to any professional's job.

If your question is: Where can I find a simple yet complete overview of the human eye and its associated disease conditions (pathology)? The answer is undoubtedly this book. The easy to read overview of the anatomy and physiology of the human eye provides excellent background knowledge. Eye pathology, like the organ it affects is also extremely complex.

This book provides an unparalleled, thorough, logical approach to eye conditions likely to be encountered and despite this book being primarily aimed at those in the beauty industry, would not be out of place in a medical library. I for one would certainly have benefited from a text like this as a medical student and junior doctor.

Dr Michael D McLaughlin MBChB FRCA

CHAPTER 1: Anatomy of the eye

The human eye is the most complex organ in the body and each component plays a significant part in how well we can see. Understanding the anatomy of the eye teaches us how to look after it, diagnose diseases and apply the necessary treatments.

How the Eye Functions

The eyes measure roughly 2.5 cm in diameter and only vary from 1-2mm between adults. The primary function of the eyes is to gather and focus light in order to transmit a clear image to light-sensitive tissues – this is the first stage of processing. The image is then transmitted to the back of the brain using electrical impulses that are sent through the optic nerves. The area of the brain which receives these electrical impulses is called the visual cortex. Here the impulses are forwarded to other parts of the brain. Fundamentally, sight is the result of electrical impulses that are delivered by the eye.

Important Tissues

Pupil

The central aperture of the iris is the pupil (the black circle). This allows light to enter the eye, but appears dark because the pigments in the retina absorb light.

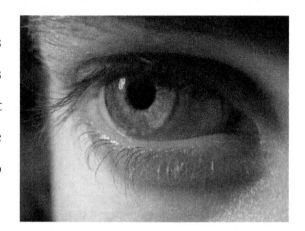

Iris

The coloured circular muscle is the iris, and is what gives the eyes their colour. The iris controls the size of the pupil so it can let in more or less light. The colour of the iris is due to variable amounts of eumelanin and pheomelanin, which is produced by melanocytes. More eumelanin results in brown eyes, while more pheomelanin results in blue or green eyes. Eumelanin and pheomelanin are types of Melanin which is a broad term for a group of natural pigments found in most organisms.

Cornea

The cornea is the transparent surface that covers the pupil and iris. The cornea is the most powerful lens of the optic system and works alongside the crystalline lens to produce sharp images.

Crystalline Lens

The crystalline lens is located directly behind the pupil and works alongside the cornea to process the incoming light. The crystalline lens automatically processes approaching objects in a process called accommodation.

Retina

The retina is the light sensitive inner lining at the back of the eye. It acts like an electronic image sensor by delivering signals to the optic nerve.

Vitreous Gel

The vitreous gel forms the main bulk of the eye and is a jelly-like substance that supports the internal structure.

Lens

The lens is a clear protein structure which helps focus images and adjusts the focusing power depending on whether the object is close or far away.

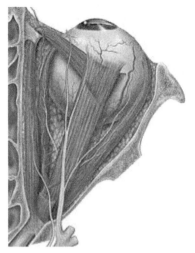

Ciliary Body

The ciliary body is a muscle which changes the shape of the lens to allow clear focusing. It is also a gland that produces a water-like substance called aqueous fluid,. This is used to keep the eyes moist.

Optic Nerve

The optic nerve is made up of fine nerve fibres that stem from the retina that exit the eye through a collection of tiny holes. These nerve fibres carry electrical impulses to the back of the brain.

Sclera

The sclera is commonly known as the white of the eye. It's a very strong opaque tissue which protects the eye's outer coat.

Extraocular Muscles

There are three (6 altogether) muscles located in the sclera. Two of the pairs, known as the superior rectus, inferior rectus, lateral rectus and medial rectus, run to the orbit of the skull. The remaining pair, are known as the superior oblique and inferior oblique, and are angled obliquely. The extraocular muscles rotate the eyeballs in the orbits and allow images to be focused onto the fovea.

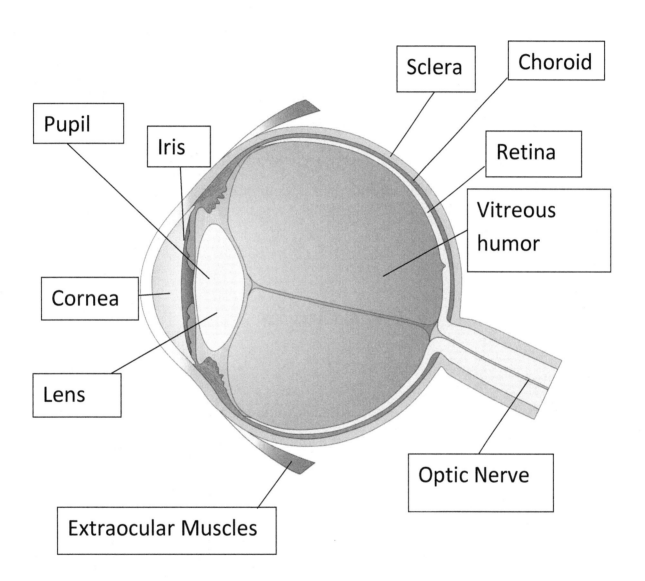

Sclera

Choroid

Pupil

Iris

Retina

Vitreous humor

Cornea

Lens

Optic Nerve

Extraocular Muscles

CHAPTER 2: Eyelash Theory

An eyelash (lash) is a hair which grows on the outer edge of the eyelid. There purpose is to protect the eye against foreign particles, parasites and chemicals. Eyelashes are located on both the upper and lower eyelids, and on each section there are between three and five layers. The eyelashes are similar to body hair and are anchored to the eyelids with a root.

Eyelash Functions

The eyelids contain small muscles that automatically contract when the eyes are subject to an external threat, such as foreign particles or chemicals; this causes blinking. When humans blink the eyelashes form a protective barrier over the eyes and release a lubricant from the sebaceous glands (tear glands) which run along the edge of the eyelids. Blinking usually occurs every seven seconds or when the eye is focusing. The lubrication ensures that the eyes don't dry out and are kept moist and healthy.

Eyelash Anatomy

Eyelashes that are located on the upper eyelid are longer than on the lower eyelid. They also tend to curve upwards and have a density of between 70 and 100 eyelashes.

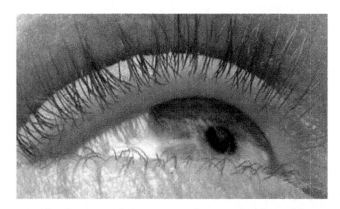

The lower eyelashes tend to curve downward and have a density of between 60 and 80 eyelashes. The curvature of the eyelashes is designed to help sweat and foreign particles flush out of the eye.

Like all human body hair, eyelashes are biological polymer and are made up from around 10 per cent water and 90 per cent protein. Proteins such as keratin and melanin give the hair its colour. Eyelashes are fed by follicles that are located just below the skin.

Eyelash Growth

Eyelashes go through three stages of hair growth:

- Anagen (active/growth phase)
- Catagen (transition/regression phase) &
- Telogen (resting phase).

Unlike hair, eyelashes and eyebrows have a very short anagen phase of about 30-45 days. The short duration of eyelash growth stage explains why they are shorter than scalp hair.

Approximately 60-80% of the eyelashes are in this phase.

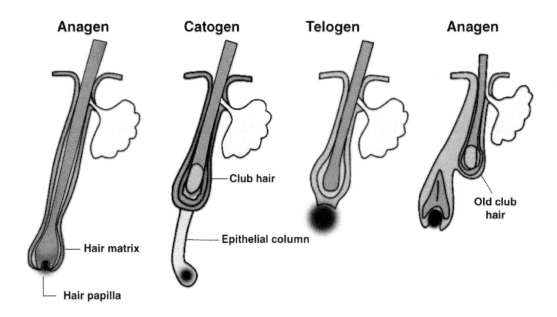

Structure of the eyelash / hair

Keratin: A protein, which forms hair.

Cuticle: The hair cuticle is the outermost part of the hair shaft

Cortex: The middle layer of hair.

Medulla: The medulla is the inner most layer of the hair shaft.
Inner Root Sheath: The inner root sheath of the hair follicle is located between the outer root sheath and the hair shaft. It is made of three layers: Henle's layer, Huxley's layer, and the cuticle.

Outer Root Sheath: The outer root sheath of the hair follicle encloses the inner root sheath and hair shaft

Connective Tissue: Connective tissue is a form of fibrous tissue. Collagen is the main protein of connective tissue.

Dermal Papillae: The dermal papillae nourishes all hair follicles and bring food and oxygen to the lower layers of epidermal cells.

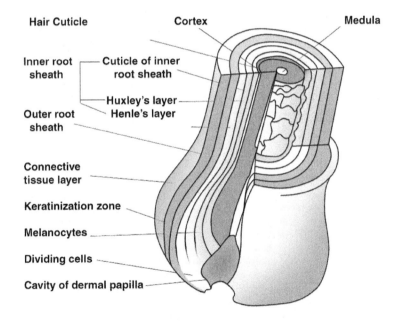

Eyelid Functions

The eyelids (palpebrae) are reinforced folds of skin which are attached to the skeletal muscles. The orbicularis oculi muscle controls the eyelids, but receives assistance from the levator palpebrae superioris muscle. The levator palpebrae superioris muscles are designated to the upper eyelid, which is why it has more freedom of movement than the lower eyelid.

CHAPTER 3: eyelash / eye diseases and disorders

When suffering from an eye disease or disorder, finding the route of the problem is the first step towards successful treatment. In most circumstances eye problems will resolve themselves after a few days and won't cause long-term damage; however, they could also be a symptom of something more serious. Early diagnosis is often essential and anyone suffering from eye related issues should always ensure they do their utmost to find out the cause.

Blepharitis

Blepharitis is the scientific term for inflammation of the eyelids. It occurs around the eyelid margins – the point where the eyelashes grow – and is caused when white blood cells and other bodily chemicals attempt to protect the eyes against foreign substances. Blepharitis can affect people of all ages; however, it is most common among those who suffer from acne and rosacea. It can also occur as a reaction to mascara, contact lens solution and airborne allergens.

Symptoms

Typical signs of Blepharitis include irritated eyelids, itching, and the formation of white specks on the eyelashes. While it can be frustrating to deal with, it's not contagious and doesn't cause permanent eye damage.

There are various forms of blepharitis:

Anterior blepharitis – eye margin inflammation.

Serborrheic blepharitis – eyelash dandruff.

Staphylococcal blepharitis – eyelash bacterial infection.

Demodex blepharitis – mite infection.

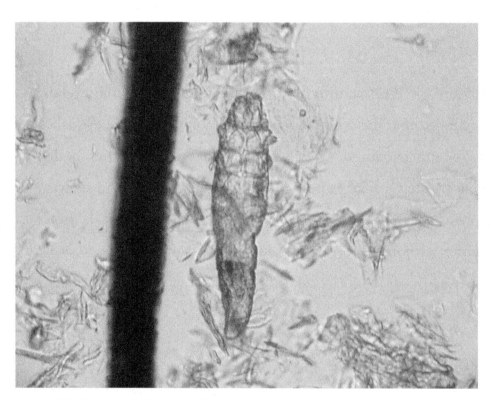

Magnified image of Demodex infection,

(Demodex mite next to hair).

Treatment

Good eyelid hygiene – such as frequent face cleaning – is the best form of prevention. Treatment methods include limiting eye makeup, using anti dandruff shampoo and temporarily avoiding contact lenses. Blepharitis usually clears up by itself within two to four weeks without any treatment; however, when symptoms continue beyond this point medical attention should be sought as long-term inflammations can lead to other issues. In extreme circumstances antibiotics may be prescribed. Researchers have found omega-3 fish oil and flaxseed supplementation beneficial in reducing symptoms.

Hordeolum / Styes

Hordeolum is a form of stye (sty) that occurs when one of the sweat glands or small sebaceous glands at the base of the eyelashes becomes blocked. This causes a bump on or inside the eyelid. Obstructions of these glands can be caused by a number of reasons such as scar tissue, makeup or dust. A hordeolum is often confused with a chalazion, which is a cyst or type of scarring that's caused by chronic inflammation of the meibomian glands.

Symptoms

The most common symptom of a hordeolum is the development of a red bump on the eyelid – similar to a pimple. Other symptoms could include discomfort when blinking, watery eyes and general tenderness. If a stye remains infected over time it may scar the meibomian gland and leave a cyst behind; however, unlike a stye, they are usually painless.

Treatment

A hordeolum should never be squeezed as this could worsen the infection; however, they can be treated at home by applying a clean, warm washcloth to the affected area for 10 minutes, four times per day. If a hordolum persists beyond three days, doctors may choose to drain it under local anaesthesia or prescribe oral antibiotics. Good eye hygiene and a diet high in omega-3 fatty acids is the best form of prevention.

Hirsutism

Hirsutism is defined by excessive hair growth in areas on a woman that are usually minimal, such as the eyebrows, upper lip and neck. In most circumstances the hair is thick and dark as opposed to fine and fair. It occurs as a result of either increased androgen production or increased androgen sensitivity. The condition is most common among women of reproductive age and the clinically obese. The specific causes of hair growth must be evaluated by a physician. They will in turn recommend the best possible treatment, be it cosmetic or medicinal.

Symptoms

The most common symptom of hirsutism is excessive hair growth; however, it's not uncommon for other symptoms to arise, such as acne, oily skin, headaches and increased libido.

Treatment

Losing weight can reduce androgen production, which reduces the effects of hirsutism. There are also various cosmetic treatments, such as laser hair removal, shaving, waxing and bleaching. In some instances oral contraceptive pills containing drospirenone are used to suppress the androgens. Flutamide is the most effective hirsutism treatment with seventeen out of eighteen women experiencing a significant reduction of abnormal hair growth when it is combined with the oral contraceptive pill.

Pseudofolliculitis

Pseudofoliculitis – also known as shaving bumps, razor bumps and barber's itch – is caused by irritations from shaving. Pseudofoliculitis most commonly occurs on the male face; however, it can affect females and any part of the body where hair can be shaved or plucked, including the eyebrows. Pseudofoliculitis is often a problem for people who have curly hair as it's caused when hair grows into the skin rather than out of the follicle. This leads to an inflammation which can make the skin turn red and cause bumps to appear.

Symptoms

Typical signs of pseudofoliculitis include redness of the skin, small bumps on the skin, itching and pimples. These small patches can cause larger, more painful pimples in the event of prolonged infection. Scar tissue may also occur as the spots heal.

Treatment

The best prevention is to allow the hair to grow out. On average, it will take pseudofoliculitis around 10 days to resolve. If the condition continues to be a problem, some doctors may choose laser-assisted hair removal to remove the follicle completely. In more severe cases where the skin becomes infected, oral antibiotics may be prescribed. If pseudofolliculitis keeps reoccurring, experimentation with shaving technique may be required. Most people find it soothing to leave a few millimetres of stubble.

Hypertrichosis

Hypertrichosis (Ambras syndrome) is condition which causes an abnormal amount of hair growth all over the body. There are two different types of hypertrichosis; generalized and localized. Generalized hypertrichosis affects the entire body, while localized is restricted to certain areas that aren't commonly associated with hair growth. Hypertrichosis rarely affects androgen-dependent areas such as the public regions, certain parts of the face and the axillary regions.

Symptoms

The most common symptom is excess hair growth which is usually longer than it should be. It may also consist of any type of hair – lanugo, vellus, terminal – even if it's not commonly found in that particular area. Some forms of hypertrichosis may grow in patterns.

Treatment

While there is no cure for hypertricosis, hair removal procedures are often used to address the issue. This could include both temporary and permanent solutions such as trimming, shaving, plucking, waxing, and laser hair removal. Hypertrichosis is often mistaken for hirsutism, which can be treated using medication that's designed to reduced androgen levels.

Folliculitis

Folliculitis is an inflammatory around the opening of the hair follicle that causes a red bump to appear. Anything from a singular to hundreds of hair follicles can be affected and it is common among teenagers who suffer from acne. Anybody can develop folliculitis – even healthy people – and it can occur wherever there is hair present on the body. While there are a variety of reasons for its formation, it's commonly caused by irritating substances such as makeup. There are various forms of folliculitis, including fungal, bacterial, viral and non-infectious. Symptoms often worsen in warm weather conditions or as a result of iron deficiency anemia.

Symptoms

The most common symptoms are numerous small red bumps. These can occur anywhere that hair grows. Sometimes the bumps can be skin coloured, which creates the appearance of 'goose bumps.' The bumps can often turn red, crusty and itchy.

Treatment

Folliculitis will usually clear up on its own without treatment. The use of over-the-counter antibacterial washes – such as benzoyl peroxide – and good skin hygiene is the best prevention method. Doctors may prescribe short term oral antibiotics; however, in most circumstances a topical antiseptic is the most effective treatment.

Ingrown hairs

Ingrown hairs are hairs which grow back into skin, rather than exiting the hair follicle. It commonly occurs when dead hair clogs up the follicle and forces it under the skin. Although ingrown hairs aren't serious, they can be irritating. Ingrown hairs produce a red bump that can sometimes look like a pimple or boil. Although anyone can get ingrown hairs, they are more common among those who have thick and curly hair,

Symptoms

Ingrown hairs most commonly occur in areas that are shaved or waxed. They usually darken the skin or cause small red bumps to appear. If they become infected these bumps can bloat into large boils where puss is collected. This can become painful and itchy.

Treatment

The best form of treatment is to wait, as ingrown hairs will eventually grow out. During this time it's important not to scratch or irritate the affected area. Not using a razor for shaving is the best form of prevention because this can cause the hair to have sharp edges which can penetrate through the skin. Steroid medicine can be used to bring down swelling and antibiotics are often prescribed in the event of an infection. If ingrown hairs continually occur, electrolysis hair removal may be required to prevent hair growth in the affected area.

Distichiasis

Distichiasis is a rare condition which causes two rows of eyelashes to grow. The extra row grows from the meibomian glands and can protrude into the cornea and cause serious corneal abrasions. There are two types of distichiasis; acquired and congenital. With acquired distichiasis, lashes form specifically on the lower eyelids. The congenital form is usually inherited.

Symptoms

Many sufferers don't have symptoms and may not even be aware of their condition. However, in most circumstances the affected eye will become red and inflamed. Some people experience the feeling of having something constantly stuck in their eye.

Treatment

It's important to treat distichiasis as soon as possible as the eyelash could scratch the surface of the eye and cause other more serious problems. Ophthalmic lubricants without preservatives can protect the cornea; however, this is only a short term solution as they must be applied between three and four times per day. Cryotherapy is often used to freeze the hair follicules to -20 degrees, which results in permanent removal. Laser treatments may also be used.

Hyperkeratosis

Hyperkeratosis is a condition which causes the thickening of the outer layer of skin. It usually occurs as a form of protection against friction, radiation from sunlight, chronic inflammations and irritating chemicals. Hyperkeratosis can occur on any part of the body and the duration can vary according to the severity. There are various different hyperkeratosis triggers, including dry air, harsh soaps, bubble baths and extreme temperatures. It can also be hereditary.

Symptoms

Typical symptoms of hyperkeratosis include corns, calluses, chronic eczema and warts. It can also occur as an allergic reaction. When hyperkeratosis frequently occurs doctors will often suggest allergy testing.

Treatment

Health care professionals can remove warts through laser removal, trimming and cryosurgery. Corns and calluses will often go with time by padding the affected area. Doctors will usually prescribe an ointment or recommend an over-the-counter medication for chronic eczema. Sometimes changing clothing may be all that's required to reduce the chance of hyperkeratosis onset, such as using cotton instead of synthetics, silk and wool.

Madarosis

Madarosis is the medical term for loss of eyelashes. It can occur for a variety of reasons, including chemical irritations, skin disorders and systematic disorders. Severe cases of madarosis can also result in a loss of eyebrows. Madarosis can also occur due to negative reactions regarding diet and cosmetic s; and in some circumstances small lifestyle changes could be all that's required to prevent it

Symptoms

Madarosis is often a side effect of other conditions such as chronic diseases of the eyelids, infections, burns, radiotherapy and chemotherapy.

The most common symptoms are partial and complete loss of eyelashes or eyebrows.

Treatment

Treatment can significantly vary according to what causes the condition. If it occurs from something cosmetic, simply preventing future application can solve the problem. Occasionally madarosis can occur as a side effect of other medications, most commonly, thyroid and blood pressure medications. Doctors will sometimes prescribe xalatan, which can promote eyelash regrowth.

Trichiasis

Trichiasis is a very common eyelid disorder that causes the eyelashes to direct towards the globe. The condition can occur across the entire lid or on a specific section. The problem is most commonly noted shortly after birth among children of Asian ancestry. Trichiasis can also form from various infections including trachoma, herpes zoster and ocular cicatricial pemphigoid.

Symptoms

Most sufferers feel like they have something stuck in their eye. This can cause itching and general discomfort that could result in corneal abrasion. Other symptoms include redness and sensitivity to bright light. Trichiasis may cause inflammations around the eye and increase the chance of infections occurring due to rubbing.

Treatment

Eye lubricants and ointments can aid comfort; however, they won't solve the problem. Lash destruction surgery and repositioning provides a more permanent solution. Azithromycin has also been known to decrease recurrence. It's important that sufferers treat trichiasis as soon as possible, otherwise other issues could occur such as conjunctivitis and corneal abrasions.

Demodex Folliculorum

Demodex folliculorum is a species of face mite that live on human hair follicles. They are often found in large quantities on the eyebrows and eyelashes and are thought to contribute to hair loss. During the day, demodex folliculorum feed on dead skin cells, while at night they emerge to the surface to mate and lay eggs. Females lay between 20 and 24 eggs in a single follicle. After they hatch it takes them seven days to mature into adults. Mites are usually between 0.1mm and 0.4mm long and are rarely harmful. Demodex mites are usually acquired at birth and almost everyone has them on their skin; however, their density usually increases with age

Symptoms

The majority of people don't suffer from any symptoms; however, the appearance of cylindrical shaped dandruff, itching and inflammations may occur. Some patients experience a burning sensation under their eyelids when the mites burrow beneath the skin.

Treatment

Lightly rubbing a cotton swab soaked in a solution containing tee tree oil and walnut oil over the eyelashes is the most effective home remedy. Mites have a lifespan of between two and three weeks, so application should occur for a minimum of this duration.

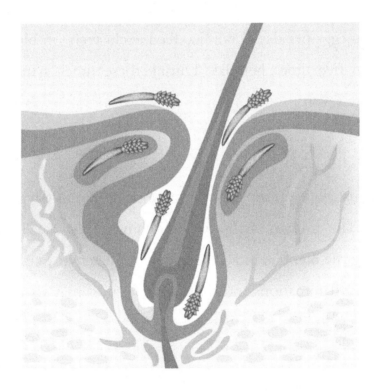

Diagram of Demodex mites surrounding hair.

Crab Lice

Crab lice (crabs) are usually found in the pubic or genital area of humans; however, they can also be found in other areas where course hair grows, such as the eyebrows and eyelashes. Crab lice are usually spread through sexual contact, but can also be transmitted through close contact of clothing, bedding and towels. Crab lice can be difficult to find because they are usually few in number. Infestation is diagnosed when eggs (nits) are found. The lifecycle of crab lice is between 16 and 25 days, and females lay around three eggs per day. Crab lice feed exclusively on blood at least four to five times per day. During these times symptoms become more severe.

Symptoms

Symptoms usually appear between five and seven days after infestation. The primary symptom is itching. This usually gets worse during the night as the lice become more active. Scratching often causes inflammations and redness. Blue spots may also occur from the biting.

Treatment

Over-the-counter shampoos and conditioners are the most common treatment. Doctors may also prescribe lindane shampoo, which is more aggressive and rarely recommended as the first line of treatment. After treatment, affected individuals should always wear clean underwear and clothing, and avoid sexual contact for at least two weeks.

Trichotillomania

Trichotillomania – also known as hair pulling disorder – is a condition which causes sufferers to pull out their hair. The average age of onset is between nine and 13 years old; and the most commonly affected areas are the scalp, eyebrows and eyelashes. People who suffer from trichotillomania usually pull out one hair at a time; and like many other psychological disorders, it can go into a state of remission for days, weeks, months or even years. It's estimated that 1.5% of males and 3.5% of females will suffer from trichotillomania at some point during their lives.

Symptoms

Trichotillomania is commonly associated with anxiety, low self-esteem, depression, obsessive compulsive disorder and post-traumatic stress syndrome. In rare instances, sufferers may also ingest their hair, which can lead to trichobezoar (hair ball) and cause digestive problems. Most sufferers will pull hair from a specific area of their scalp; however, eyelashes, eyebrows, face, arms and legs are also common pulling sites.

Treatment

Treatment will significantly vary depending on the individual's age and whether or not it occurs as a result of another underlying condition. Most children will grow out of the condition, while adults may have to undertake psychotherapy or could be prescribed medication such as a tricyclic antidepressant.

Trichophagia

Trichophagia is a more extreme version of trichotillomania (hair pulling) where sufferers ingest hair that they pull. In most circumstances individuals will eat the root bulb of their hair rather than their shaft itself. Eventually hair can accumulate in the gastrointestinal tract and cause serious medical problems. Although most sufferers consume hair from their scalp, some will ingest hair from other areas such as their eyelashes and eyebrows.

Symptoms

Ritual tasting and chewing of hair is the most common symptom. While most symptoms are psychological, in more extreme instances trichophagia can cause stomach pains and nutritional deficiencies.

Treatment

Like trichotillomania, treatment varies according to the age of the patient and their general health. Psychotherapy is the most common treatment. If the condition develops into rapunzel syndrome, which occurs when a trichobezoar (hair ball) reaches the intestines, surgery may be required to remove the mass. In some instances the mass of hair can protrude into the intestines and be fatal.

Alopecia

Alopecia is a hair loss condition. While it usually affects the scalp, it can also affect the eyebrows and eyelashes as well. Hair loss may be total or partial and could occur due to other medical conditions or as a side effect to unrelated medications or chemotherapy. Hormonal imbalances are the most common cause. Sometimes the disease will have alternating periods of hair loss and growth.

Symptoms

Alopecia is generally a symptom of another underlying condition, be it a physical, psychological or medicinal issue. Eyebrow alopecia doesn't always cause a complete loss of eyebrow hair, it can also cause thinning and spot boldness.

Treatment

Treatment for alopecia will vary depending on the underlying cause. In most circumstances the condition stems from autoimmune disorders. Treatment rarely revolves around alopecia itself; however, when treating alopecia directly, anti-inflammatory steroids are often applied to the affected area or injected into the patient. This can suppress immune reaction that attacks hair follicles, which allows them to recover. If the condition is psychological, psychiatric treatment may be the best course of action.

Conjunctivitis

CONJUNCTIVITIS

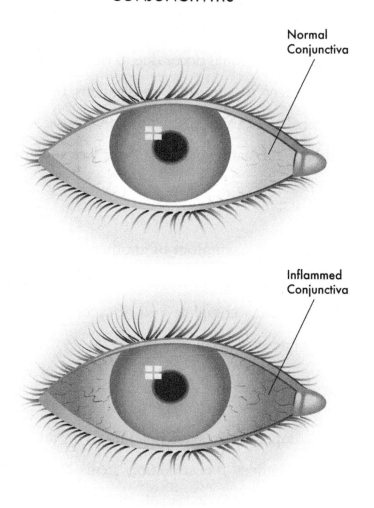

Normal Conjunctiva

Inflammed Conjunctiva

Conjunctivitis (pink eye) is an inflammation of the conjunctiva and usually occurs due to an infection or allergic reaction. There are many different forms of conjunctivitis, each with their own symptoms. Classification is usually based upon the extent of the inflammation. GP's often diagnose conjunctivitis through eye examinations; however, when symptoms continue after treatment, they may require swab tests in order to effectively diagnose the problem.

Symptoms

The most common symptom is the swelling of the conjunctiva, red eye and excessive watering. These are coherent across all classifications. Conjunctivitis shouldn't affect visual acuity.

Treatment

The best form of prevention is good general hygiene and preventing hand-to-eye contact, as this could cause an infection. In most circumstances symptoms will naturally resolve themselves after two to five days; however, if they don't, doctors may prescribe antibiotics. Contact lenses or eye makeup should not be worn during a spell of conjunctivitis as they could prolong the problem and make the symptoms worse.

Bacterial conjunctivitis

Bacterial conjunctivitis is an infection of the conjunctiva. It is a fairly common condition and rarely causes serious eye morbidity. The bacteria is often spread between affected individuals, therefore, poor hygiene is often the cause. Foreign objects such as makeup and contact lenses increase the chance of a bacterial infection. Typically, symptoms will occur on one eye and then spread to the other.

Symptoms

Symptoms usually last for between two and five days and include redness, irritation, burning and decreased vision. Some suffers will also have a stringy yellow discharge and severe crusting on the surrounding skin. Symptoms are said to feel gritty, as if something is stuck in the eye.

Treatment

In most circumstances bacterial conjunctivitis will naturally clear within 10 days; however, doctors often prescribe antibiotics in order to speed up eradication and ease the duration of symptoms. Good general hygiene and regular hand washing is the best prevention. Many doctors will recommend the "watch and wait" method. This revolves around keeping an eye on the condition for one week, and if there's no improvement, seeking medical attention. If treatment is prescribed, it should be continued for at least two days after the symptoms have subsided.

Viral conjunctivitis

Viral conjunctivitis is often associated with the common cold and flu. A typical sign of viral conjunctivitis is a pinkness of the conjunctiva. The condition rarely occurs by itself and is almost always a symptom of upper respiratory tract infections. Symptoms of viral conjunctivitis can be more severe than other forms.

Symptoms

The most common symptoms include excessive watering, redness and itching. Since viral conjunctivitis is usually a symptom of the cold and flu, sufferers may also have a runny nose, sore throat or headache. Symptoms usually last for between two and three weeks and will often get a lot worse before they get better.

Treatment

Strict hygiene management is paramount during a spell of viral conjunctivitis and patients must not share towels or go swimming, otherwise they could infect others. The condition doesn't have any form of specific treatment and will clear up by itself when the cold or flu subsides; however, antihistamines and vitamin C intake may ease symptoms and reduce their duration.

Chlamydial conjunctivitis

Chlamydial conjunctivitis (trachoma) is one of the most common causes of blindness. The infection can be spread through sexual contact, towel sharing, touching the eye, clothes, coughing and sneezing. Newborns could also become affected during childbirth. By 2020 the International Coalition of Trachoma Control plans to complete eradicate the infection worldwide. A single acute infection of chlamydial conjunctivitis is not considered sight threatening; however, ocular complications, including blindness can occur if it's left untreated.

Symptoms

Symptoms include roughening of the eyelids, sticky discharge, crusting of the lashes and surrounding skin, glued eyelids, redness, irritations, sensitivity to light and blurred vision. Some sufferers don't suffer from any symptoms and the severity can drastically change between each person.

Treatment

Chlamydial conjunctivitis is treated using two different forms of antibiotics: a pill that is ingested orally and kills the infection, and an eye drop or ointment. Symptoms will usually clear up within a few days, but could take up to one month until they are completely gone. Chlamydial conjunctivitis should not be left untreated and sufferers should always inform previous sexual partners if they are infected. Safe sex and good general hygiene is the best form of prevention.

Allergic conjunctivitis

Allergic conjunctivitis is commonly caused by pollen allergies during the hay fever season; however, it can also occur from dust mites, cosmetics and issues with contact lenses. Allergies occur when the body's immune system over-reacts to something which causes inflammations. There are various types of allergic conjunctivitis, each classified by the reaction trigger:

Seasonal – pollen, mould

Perennial – house dust mites and animals

Giant papillary – contact lenses

Contact – cosmetics, eye drops and chemicals

Symptoms

With allergic conjunctivitis symptoms tend to develop much faster than other forms. The white parts of the eye will often turn red or pink, and the eyelids may swell. In most circumstances the eyes will also become more watery and/or gluey. In more severe circumstances sensitivity to bright lights and general eye pain could occur.

Treatment

If symptoms are mild, no treatment is necessary and in many instances they will subside within a matter of hours. Eye drops and antihistamines are the most common form of treatment; however, in severe cases, steroid eye drops and tablets may be prescribed. Staying away from the irritant is the best form of prevention. Allergy tests may be required in order to discover what's triggering the condition.

Reactive conjunctivitis – chemical or irritant conjunctivitis

Reactive conjunctivitis is caused by chemicals and irritants such as chlorine in swimming pools, smoke fumes and contact lens solution.

Like other forms of conjunctivitis, it causes inflammations of the conjunctiva when triggered and isn't sight threatening.

Symptoms

Symptoms of reactive conjunctivitis can vary depending on the individual and irritant; however, in most circumstances redness, swelling and excessive watering will occur.

Treatment

Symptoms will usually subside quickly, sometimes within a matter of hours. While reactive conjunctivitis doesn't usually need treatment, doctors may recommend over-the-counter eye drops or antihistamines to relieve symptoms. Avoiding the irritant is the best prevention.

Cataract

CATARACT

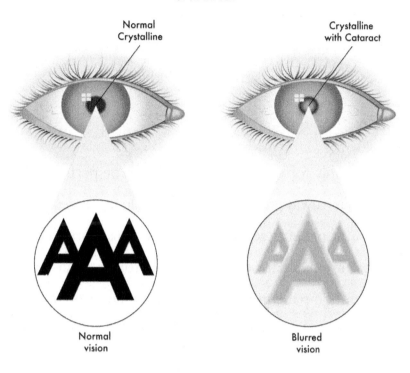

Cataract is a condition which leads to a clouding of the eye lens. This causes blurred vision and is one of the most common causes of blindness. Cataract occurs when light is obstructed from passing the lens and reaching the retina. The most common cause of cataract is ageing; however, it can also occur as a result of trauma, radiation, genetics and drug use. People who suffer from cataract often have trouble driving, reading and recognizing others.

Symptoms

Cataract affects the eyes in many ways. Some sufferers don't experience blurred vision, but find it difficult to recognise certain colours, changes in contrast and glare from bright lights. Symptoms that could occur after surgery include retinal detachment and endophthalmitis. In these cases, patients will often experience pain and will become more sensitive to bright lights.

Treatment

Surgery is the only form of treatment and can be performed at any age. Surgery is always conducted under local anaesthesia and roughly 90% of patients regain full vision. Phacoemulsification is the most common form of surgery used for cataract treatment. After an operation patients must not strain their eyes or undertake heavy lifting for around one month. There is currently no known prevention method for cataract apart from weak evidence to suggest that vitamin A, B and C could help.

Corneal Disease

Corneal disease directly affects the cornea – the clear tissue in the front of the eye which allows light to pass through to the retina. Corneal disease either affects the clarity or curvature of the cornea, which results in blurred vision. It can be caused through infections, trauma, autoimmune disorders, genetics and inflammatory diseases.

Symptoms

Corneal disease can cause severe pain if the cornea is torn as it can affect nearby nerves. The most common symptoms include sensitivity to light, irritation and blurred vision.

Treatment

Treatment for corneal disease will vary depending on the underlying condition. In some circumstances surgery may be required, while in others laser eye treatment or prescription antibiotics may suffice. Good general hygiene and regular vaccinations are the best preventative measures. Sunglasses with 100% ultraviolet block will also minimize damage from the sun's rays, and diets heavy in omega-3 fatty acids are also recommended.

Diabetic retinopathy

Diabetic retinopathy is a common condition associated with diabetes, and if it's left untreated it can result in blindness. Diabetic retinopathy is caused by high blood sugar levels which damage the cells in the eye. The retina requires a constant supply of blood, which is fed through small blood vessels. High blood sugar can cause these vessels to block or leak, which stops the retina from working. Scientists state that 90% of diabetic retinopathy cases could be reduced if patients had more frequent eye checks. The longer people suffer from diabetes, the higher the chance they'll have of suffering from diabetic retinopathy. Almost all patients that have been suffering from type I diabetes for over 20 years have some degree of the condition.

Symptoms

Anyone who suffers from diabetes should have their eyes regularly examined; symptoms may not occur until it's too late, so it's important that it's identified and treated as soon as possible. Late stage symptoms could include floaters, blurred vision and sudden blindness.

Treatment

Treatment of diabetic retinopathy will vary depending on the stage it has reached. If caught early it can be treated through correct diabetes management. When it has reached advanced stages, laser eye surgery can be used to prevent further damage. The best preventative measure is to have regular screenings and keep blood sugar levels as normal as possible.

Dry eye syndrome

Dry eye syndrome, also known as dry eye disease, occurs when either the eyes don't make enough tears or the tears evaporate too quickly. The condition leads to inflamed and irritated eyes. If it is caused by a blockage of the oil glands, it's called blepharitis. There are a number of different causes, such as hot and windy climates, hormonal changes, medication side effects and aging. It's rarely a serious condition, unless it has been caused by an inflammation or problem associated with another disease.

Symptoms

Dry and sore eyes are the most common symptoms. Blurred vision, heavy watering, grittiness and burning can also occur. Symptoms will often get worse in warmer conditions and prolonged dry eye syndrome can significantly increase the chance of other eye disorders from occurring. Severe symptoms may also be a side effect of cornea scarring.

Treatment

Dry eye syndrome must be treated straight away; otherwise it could cause permanent eye damage. Eye drops are the most common form of treatment as they will provide the lost lubrication. Surgery may be required to block drainage tear ducts which cause leakages. There are various forms of prevention and after-treatment, including using a humidifier to moisten the air, not sitting in front of a fire, avoiding eye strain from computers or television screens, and having a diet high in omega-3 fatty acids.

Glaucoma

Glaucoma is a category of conditions which affects vision, often in both eyes on varying levels. It is caused by blockages in the drainage ducts, which prevents fluid from flushing efficiently. The pressure caused by this excess fluid can damage the optic nerve and retina. There are four primary types of glaucoma:

Chronic open-angle glaucoma – this usually develops slowly with age and is the most common form.

Primary angle-closure glaucoma – this often causes sudden pains and can develop either slowly or suddenly.

Secondary glaucoma – this is often caused by other eye conditions and inflammations.

Developmental glaucoma – this usually develops soon after birth and can be very serious.

Symptoms

Most cases of glaucoma don't present any symptoms as it usually develops slowly. The first part of the eye to be affected is the peripheral vision, after which, it slowly works its way to the centre. Other symptoms could include intense pain, headaches, tenderness, misty vision, light sensitivity and loss of vision. Typical progression to blindness usually takes between 25 to 70 years without any treatment.

Treatment

Treatment revolves around reducing pressure in the eye. This could include switching to glasses instead of using contact lenses, using prescription eye drops, laser treatment and surgery to remove the blockage. Pressure can also be treated with eye drops. While these treatments can provide a temporary solution, none of them will solve the problem permanently as there is currently no cure.

Herpes simplex

Herpes simplex eye infections are caused by the herpes simplex virus. Although in most circumstances it will clear up without treatment, it can cause scarring of the cornea and lead to permanent loss of vision if left untreated. Herpes simplex will affect at least one in 1,000 people and usually becomes active between the ages of 30 and 40. Most people who suffer from the condition have had other forms of herpes in the past, such as cold sores. The virus will often go into remission and then suddenly cause breakouts that usually last for between two and 21 days.

Symptoms

It can be difficult to diagnose herpes simplex because reactions can occur years after primary infection. Common symptoms include redness, pains and aches, excessive watering and blurred vision.

Treatment

Before medication is prescribed an eye specialist must scrape away affected cells from the surface of the patient's eye. They will then numb the eye through a procedure called debridement. Antiviral eye drops are then applied; and while they do not eradicate the virus, they prevent it from multiplying. Application of the eye drops are usually made several times per day over the course of two weeks. Because herpes simplex can be transmitted through sexual contact, condoms are the best form of prevention and can reduce the chance of contracting the virus by 30%. Once somebody is infected with the herpes virus they have it for life; however, over time outbreaks will decrease in frequency and severity.

Watery eyes

Watery eyes are defined by an excessive amount of tears flowing from the eyes. Is occurs when there are either problems with eye drainage or too much tear production. It's often a side effect of other eye conditions, such as conjunctivitis or blepharitis.

When people blink, tears are spread over the surface of the globe and then pass into channels named canaliculi. They in turn drain into the tear sac and run down the side of the nose. Watery eyes are the result of problems associated with this process.

Symptoms

Watery eyes are most commonly a symptom of an existing eye disorder. The extent of tear production can vary significantly depending on the individual and their condition. Prolonged symptoms can cause soreness around the eyes due to excessive rubbing.

Treatment

Treatment of the underlying issue is usually preferred. If a sufferer only has watery eyes, treatment may not be necessary at all as the problem will often resolve itself over time. In the event of a blocked tear duct, surgery may be required. Good general face and eye hygiene is the best prevention method. Sufferers should not rub their eyes, as this could prolong the problem and cause infections.

If watery eyes are caused by another eye condition such as conjunctivitis, antibiotics may be prescribed.

Eye infection

Eye infections occur when harmful microorganisms invade the eyes or eyelids. This could include bacteria, fungi and viruses. There are many different types of eye infections, each with varying levels of severity. Sufferers should always book an appointment to have an eye exam if they suspect that they have an infection because early treatment is often paramount in order to prevent long-term damage. Conjunctivitis is the most common eye infection and is highly contagious; therefore, in the event of contracting an eye infection, patients should maintain an excellent level of general hygiene and should not share towels, clothes or make close contact with others.

Symptoms

Eye infections can cause anything from mild symptoms such as watering, redness and itching; to serious symptoms such as blurred vision, severe pains and loss of vision. Eye infections can be very serious if they are left undiagnosed.

Treatment

Treatment will significantly vary depending on the age of the patient, their condition and how long their eye has been infected. Doctors may need to take a sample of the infected cells in order to pinpoint the cause of the infection and provide the best possible treatment. Most infections may be left alone to cure by themselves; however, others may require a course of antibiotics or even surgery. The best way to prevent eye infections is through good hygiene and hand washing.

Atopic Eczema / Atopic dermatitis

Atopic eczema is the most common form of eczema. The condition causes skin to become itchy, dry, red and cracked. While atopic eczema is most common among children, it can affect sufferers into adulthood. Atopic eczema often occurs around the eyes and can vary in severity. While to most sufferers it's nothing but an inconvenience, to some it can cause serious pain and bleeding. The cause of atopic eczema is still unknown; however, it's more common among those who suffer from allergies and has been known to be hereditary.

Symptoms

Typical symptoms include dry, cracked, flaky and itchy skin. This can occur anywhere on the body, but is most commonly found around the eyes, behind the knees, inside the elbows, on the ears and on the side of the neck. Sufferers will often have periods when symptoms clear up, and others when the outbreaks are more severe. Symptoms may also only occur when the affected area is exposed to an irritant, such as a fabric or chemical that causes allergies.

Treatment

In most circumstances symptoms of atopic eczema will clear with age, and in 53% of circumstances, it completely clears by the time children reach the age of 11. The main form of treatment includes emollients (moisturiser) and topical corticosteroids. This can reduce swelling and pain during severe flare-ups. There is currently no evidence to suggest that oral antibiotics have any positive effects, so they are only prescribed if the condition is causing other problems.

Psoriasis

Psoriasis is a common skin condition which often affects the eyelids. It causes patches of red, scaly skin to appear, which can feel dry and flaky. It occurs when the top layer of skin is flattened and sheds off, which causes the basal layer to replace the top layer. The extent of the rash varies between different people. While some may only have one small patch measuring a few millimetres, others may have patches that are inches across. Chronic psoriasis can be itchy; however, it's not known to cause too much discomfort. Roughly one in 50 people develop psoriasis at some point in their life, usually between the ages of 15 and 30.

Symptoms

Typical symptoms include dry skin, itchy skin, flaky skin and redness. Outbreaks can also result in mobility pains if the rash flares up on skin located over a joint. At least 30% of psoriasis sufferers also experience psoriatic arthritis. Symptoms can also occur as a side effect of medicines and psychological disorders.

Treatment

Because the cause is not understood and is generally passed on genetically, psoriasis is a difficult condition to treat. Smoking, excessive exposure to sunlight, lack of sleep, weight and stress significantly increases risk and sometimes tackling these issues is all that's required to relieve symptoms. While there is no cure for psoriasis, emollients and vitamin D based treatments are available to help sooth pain and ease symptoms. Steroid creams may also be prescribed in order to reduce inflammations. Omega-3 fatty acids and cod liver oil may provide dietary benefits.

Macular Degeneration

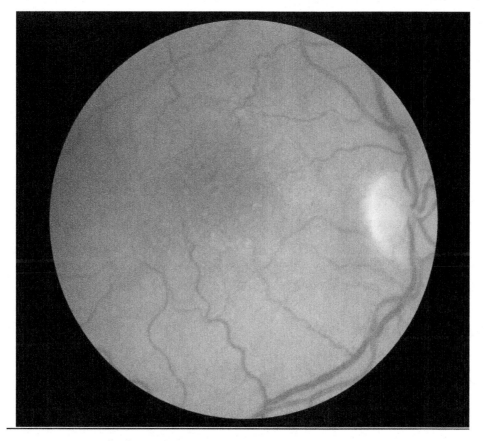

A Fundus photo showing Macular Degeneration.

Macular degeneration is a painless eye condition which usually occurs with age. It causes vision to become increasingly blurry and makes colours appear less vibrant. Because it doesn't affect peripheral vision, it can't cause a complete loss of sight. While macular degeneration usually affects both eyes, the speed of progression can significantly vary. Loss of vision is very slow and usually occurs over the course of many years. It's currently the leading cause of visual impairment in the UK and tends to be more common among women than men.

Symptoms

All macular degeneration symptoms are related to quality of sight. Blurred vision and difficulty distinguishing faces are the most common issues. In serious occurrences, blind spots or hallucinations may also occur directly in the middle of the visual field. Less serious symptoms usually occur between five and 10 years before visuals are affected. These include sensitivity to light, colours appearing less vibrant and hazy outbreaks. When symptoms develop, medical treatment should be sought at the earliest possible convenience.

Treatment

There is currently no cure for macular degeneration. Treatment usually revolves around helping individual's make the most out of the vision they have with glasses and contact lenses. Some evidence suggests that consumption of leafy green vegetables can prolong macular degeneration. Early diagnosis is often essential when preventing severe loss of vision as the condition can be treated with ani-VEGF medication; this stops it from getting worse. In some instances laser eye surgery can be used to destroy abnormal blood vessels.

Flashes and Floaters

Flashes and floaters are very common and can occur either together or separately. They are often a complaint among the elderly and are usually attributed to the collapse of vitreous gel. However, there are also more serious causes as well, such as retinal detachment.

Flashes (photopsia) occur when the individual sees flashing lights – like a lightbulb switching on and off in quick succession. They are primarily caused by two reasons; improper stimulation of the retina and problems with the optic nerve.

Floaters are opacities that float in the sufferer's field of vision. They are usually seen as spots or wavy lines. They move with eye movements and will often disperse when the patient looks at them directly. There are a number of causes for floaters such as ageing, vitreous detachment, inflammatory cells and tumours. In around 25% of circumstances, no underlying causes are found. Most people tend to ignore floaters and get used to them after time.

Symptoms

Typical symptoms of flashes include seeing lights, stars and halos. While symptoms of floaters usually revolve around seeing shapes, they can lead to headaches when the patient focuses on them.

Treatment

In most circumstances flashes and floaters won't require any treatment and will fade over the course of time. Vitamin therapy may cause them to disappear, however, even this is rarely recommended. Vitreous floaters may be caused by a tear in the retina; this may require surgery to prevent the retina from detaching from the eye.

Allergic Reactions

Allergic reactions in the eye are often more irritating than dangerous and won't cause long-term damage. The most common causes of allergic reactions are hay fever and atopic eczema. Medications and cosmetics could also have a significant affect. The triggers behind these causes are usually pollen, dust mites, moulds and household pets.

Allergic reactions can affect anybody of any age. They can also lie dormant for many years or return on a seasonal basis. In some instances they occur early in life and relieve themselves with age.

Symptoms

Typical symptoms are akin to the flu and common cold, such as swelling, heavy watering, red eyes, and inflammation of the conjunctiva. Most sufferers will feel the urge to rub their eyes; however, this can only prolong the problem and make it worse.

Treatment

Antihistamines are the most common treatments and can be taken either in pill form or as an eye drop. Oral medications such as loratadine and cetirizine are generally less effective than eye drops when treating eye conditions.

During particularly bad outbreaks, doctors may prescribe a topical steroid to relieve symptoms on a short-term basis.

CHAPTER 4: Taking care of the eye area

The eyes are a fragile and sensitive part of the human body and learning how to minimize risk is a crucial aspect of healthy living.

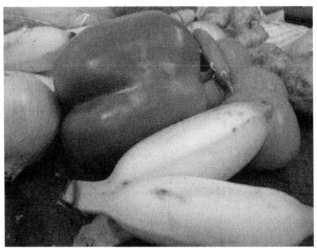

In many cases, eye problems and disorders can be prevented, and simple hygiene and dietary practices could be all that's required to keep them in good standing. Although some eye conditions are caused by other underlying medical problems, taking good care of the eyes can reduce symptoms and help sufferers lead a more comfortable lifestyle.

Diet and Nutrition

Diet and nutrition plays a huge part in the general health of the eyes. Those who have diets rich in fruit, vegetables and omega-3 fatty acids will be much less likely to suffer from eye conditions. Vitamins A, C and E are of particular benefit, as they contain vital antioxidants that can significantly reduce damage occurring to the retina and lens. This can protect the eyes from age related disorders such as cataract and macular degeneration.

Spinach, squash, tomatoes, corn, broccoli, carrots, turnip, sprouts and cabbage are highly recommended. Reducing salt intake can also decrease blood pressure, which is one of the fundamental problems behind a number of eye conditions.

Alcohol and Smoking

Excessive consumption of alcohol can cause gradual loss of vision, making colours appear paler with less contrast. Smoking has been known to speed up age related macular degeneration, which can significantly affect reading vision. Tobacco smoking can also cause the surface of the eye to dry out, leaving it itchy and irritated. This increases the risk of infection as most sufferers will rub their eyes in an attempt to sooth symptoms. Over any other form of general health practice, quitting smoking and reducing alcohol intake is the best preventative measure that smokers and heavy drinkers can take.

Exercise

Exercise will significantly improve the cardiovascular system. Improving blood flow around the eye will significantly hinder the onset of issues associated with blood pressure such as blockages. In addition, it can also reduce the risk of type-2 diabetes, which can also lead to visual impairment.

At least 30 minutes of medium intensity exercise, four to five times per week is recommended in order to maintain good health. Such exercises include jogging, cycling and rowing. Making simple lifestyle changes can also be of benefit, such as taking the stairs instead of the lift or walking to work instead of driving.

Sun Exposure

Excessive exposure to ultraviolet light (UV) from the sun can burn the cornea. This can also occur from tanning equipment. Skiers will often suffer from this problem due to the suns reflection off snow, which is why the condition is often referred to as "snow blindness." Staring directly at the sun can cause permanent damage to sight. Simple preventative measures can be taken, such as applying sun screen to the face and around the eyes, and wearing sunglasses.

Eye Protection

Eyeglasses should never be used for safety. When working around power tools or in an area that has a large accumulation of loose debris, safety goggles must be worn. Eyeglasses don't protect a very large surface area, so it's easy for foreign objects to find their way around the lenses. In addition, shards of glass could pose an ever greater risk if they are broken.

Regular Checkups

Most people will wait until there is an issue before they see a medical professional; however, there's no better preventative measure than having regular checkups.

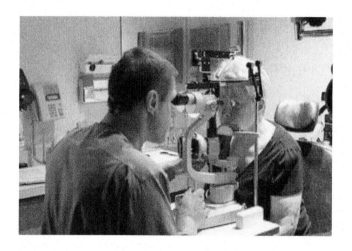

Catching eye problems early is often the key to successful treatment. At least one checkup every two to four years is recommended for those below 65; and one check-up every one to two years for those above 65. People who suffer from short-sightedness should take more frequent screenings than others.

General Eye Care Facts

- Watching television in a dark room can cause excess strain on the eyes.

- Dim light is easier for reading, but can result in tiredness.

- Frequent breaks are recommended from anything that requires significant eye strain. This will give the muscles time to relax.

- Monitors, televisions and books should be placed at eye level or just below.

- Anti-glare filters are highly recommended for those who regularly work on a computer.

- Glasses and contacts will significantly reduce eye strain.

General Eye Treatment

Minor eye injuries will often clear up by themselves and will rarely require medical treatment. However, an appointment with a GP should always be arranged in the event of:

- Persistent eye pains.

- Pain looking at bright lights.

- Disturbances with vision.

- Continual redness.

- Foreign objects that can't be washed out

In some instances, when the eyes are subject to a severe infection or trauma, referral to an eye specialist may be required. Such occurrences include:

- Injuries caused by high-speed flying objects.

- Injuries caused by corrosive chemicals.

- Foreign objects that can't be washed out by a GP.

- Severe eye pains.

- Severe disturbances or deterioration of vision.

- Deep cuts on the orbit.

- Recurring minor injuries or infections.

- Injuries that fail to improve after general treatment.

When treatment is needed, daily examinations by an eye specialist may be required until the eye has fully healed.

Eye and Facial Hygiene

Bacteria, dirt and other foreign particles that are stuck to the face can often pass through the eyelids and come into contact with the surface of the eye. Anything from dirty clothes to fine crumbs from the kitchen can cause this problem, and exposure to the eyes' surface will often lead to irritations and infections. Good general hygiene is the best way to prevent these problems from occurring.

How to Safely Wash Your Eyes

Eyes are extremely sensitive organs that can be easily irritated. Small minute particles, invisible to the naked eye can cause a significant level of discomfort and lead to infections. While natural tearing can flush particles out of the eye, there are occasions when human intervention is required.

Directions:

Before you try to flush out any foreign particles, try to make yourself cry by blinking. Sometimes getting the tears to flow is all that's required.

Step One

Always conduct the cleaning process in a well-lit, sanitized area in the bathroom by washing the surfaces with antibacterial cleaner and warm water.

Step Two

Wash your hands thoroughly with warm water and antibacterial soap prior to touching the affected eye. Failure to take this precautionary measure could result in infections.

Step Three

Inspect your eyes under the light to determine the nature and position of the irritant.

Step Four

Clean an eye dropper, egg cup or small glass with warm water and antibacterial soap. Make sure it's been thoroughly rinsed before continuing. Fill it with clean cool water.

Step Five

Hold your upper eyelid up, away from the eye and place the cool water over your open eye. Try to flush out the particle by rolling your eyes. Repeat this process until you can no longer feel the irritant.

Step Six

Inspect your eye to ensure it's been removed.

Warnings:

- If you can't remove the particle, ask somebody to drive you to the emergency room as soon as possible. Do not try to remove it with your fingers, otherwise you could infect the eye or scratch the cornea, which could lead to further complications.

- Never put anything besides water inside your eye.

- If the particle is embedded, do not try to remove it without professional medical assistance.

Tips:

- Always wash your face at least twice per day with warm water and mild soap. Gently massage your face in a circular motion and don't scrub too hard as this could cause your skin to become irritated. Using an over-the-counter lotion such as benzoyl peroxide will decrease oil and bacteria and reduce the risk of infection.

- Do not pop pimples, otherwise the infected fluid could get into your eyes and cause further damage.

- After cleaning your face try to avoid touching it with your fingers. Sebum and other foreign particles will often collect on objects such as your phone and television remote. Touching your face can spread bacteria from these objects and cause infections.

- If you wear glasses or sunglasses, make sure you clean them frequently to prevent the oil that gets collected on them from clogging your pores around your nose and eyes.

- Always remove makeup before you go to sleep and throw away makeup that smells or looks different to when you first purchased it.

- Wash your hair regularly and keep it out of your face to prevent oil and dirt clogging your pores and getting into your eyes.

Soothing Symptoms

Quickly eradicating symptoms isn't always possible; however, there is a technique of applying warmth and massage that can help relieve certain problems and encourage blocked meibomian glands to clear of any oily secretions..

The purpose of applying warmth is to soften the skin and the crusts around the eyelids. It will also encourage secretions from the meibomian glands to become runny and flow more freely.

Warmth

This three step process is a daily routine that consists of warmth, massage and cleansing.

Step one – soak a clean flannel in warm water.

Step two – press the flannel against your eyelids for five to ten minutes.

Step three – re-soak the flannel in warm water again if it gets cold and repeat the process.

Massage

The massage phase should be conducted immediately after application of warmth. This will help push out oily fluid.

Step one – place your index or middle finger on the corner of your eye next to your nose. Gently sweep your finger above the upper lashes to the outer end of your eyelid.

Step two – place your index or middle finger on the corner of your eye next to your nose. Gently sweep your finger below the lower lashes towards your temple.

Step three – repeat the sweeping motion about five to ten times within a one minute period. Apply as much pressure as feels comfortable and soothing.

Cleansing

Cleansing will remove any excess fluid that has collected on your face and nose.

Step one – wash your hands with warm water and antibacterial soap to remove any dirt or fluid which has collected during the massage phase.

Step two – rinse your face with warm water and then immediately apply an antibacterial face wash.

Step three – thoroughly rinse off the soap with clean warm water, and then dry your face with a clean towel.

Thank you for purchasing and reading this book, I hope you found it useful.

For further information in the books we produce or if you would like to submit a title for publication please contact us publishinguk@icloud.com

CPSIA information can be obtained
at www.ICGtesting.com
Printed in the USA
LVOW02s1527120116
470291LV00013B/734/P

9 781500 657093